THE ULTIMATE GUIDE TO STRAIGHTENING YOUR SMILE

(So You Can Look Fabulous)

— An Orthodontist Mom's Secret Recipes for Using Braces and Invisalign®

Published by CelebrityPress®, Orlando, FL

CelebrityPress® is a registered trademark.

Printed in the United States of America.

ISBN: 978-0-9966887-7-2
LCCN: 2016933703

CelebrityPress®
520 N. Orlando Ave, #2
Winter Park, FL 32789
or call 1.877.261.4930

Visit us online at: www.CelebrityPressPublishing.com

THE ULTIMATE GUIDE TO STRAIGHTENING YOUR SMILE

(So You Can Look Fabulous)

— An Orthodontist Mom's Secret Recipes for Using Braces and Invisalign®

By

Victoria Chen, DDS, MS

CONTENTS

INTRODUCTION

Hi, my name is Victoria Chen. For the past fifteen years, I have been working relentlessly to create the most fabulous smiles for kids, adolescents, and adults with braces and Invisalign®. My goal is to use the simplest treatment methods and devices to transform your smile in the shortest period of time. I firmly believe that everyone can be a superstar! Our goal is to create your fabulous Superstar Smile for a lifetime.

I have treated thousands of patients, and I notice that some people perceive orthodontic treatment as an elective cosmetic procedure. Yes, unlike heart disease or terminal cancers, you WILL NOT DIE if you don't treat crooked teeth or smiles. You can always justify that crooked teeth or smiles will not affect your overall health, social status and self-esteem. *The truth is, crooked teeth and smiles are chronic diseases and symbols of "indifference" and "low social economic status."*

I am proud of being a mother and a female orthodontist. Also, I consider myself one of the most honest orthodontists on Earth! I myself am a mother of two young girls. I, just like all the busy and dedicated mothers and parents like you, need to decide on the best schools, afterschool programs, teachers, coaches, dentists and doctors for my own kids. As a mother, I am strong-willed, and only want to work with the "best-of-the-best" for my beloved daughters. I want to make sure that all the professionals interacting with my children are trustworthy and honest, and will take excellent care of my children. I know how scared a mother can feel to hand their loved ones over to somebody without building the "trust" factor. Therefore, as a mother and orthodontist, I know how you feel, moms and parents.

My goal is to give you my honest opinion and complete information you need to know about braces and Invisalign®, and how to achieve that lifetime **Fabulous Superstar Smile** for your children, yourself, and your family! I promise you that all the information and philosophies I recommend in this book is being, or will be, utilized on my own daughters and my patients, whom I treat as my own family.

Let's get your Fabulous Superstar Smile journey started!

N.B. This book is not for parents or patients who only want their crooked teeth fixed with the "cheapest orthodontist!" Good orthodontists are not cheap! If you are only looking for the "discount way" to fix your smiles for a lifetime, please stop reading and give this book to somebody else! No offense, I just do not want to waste your precious time.

CHAPTER 1

HOW DO I CHOOSE THE RIGHT ORTHODONTIST?
— ARE THERE DIFFERENCES AMONG ORTHODONTISTS?

WHAT IS AN ORTHODONTIST?

It is a very long, competitive process to become a licensed orthodontist. After graduating from an undergraduate college, one will then go to dental school for four years and you have to be in the top 1% of the students in dental school to apply for orthodontic programs. The orthodontic programs are very limited and selective in the United States! It takes another 2-3 more years for the dentists to become orthodontists. All orthodontists are dentists, but only 5% of dentists are orthodontists.

An orthodontist can diagnose and treat the following problems that most family dentists may not:

    a. Protruding front teeth

    b. Deep bite or underbite

    c. Teeth erupting the wrong way so that they do not overlap together (openbite)

    d. Crowding, impacted, or malformed teeth

    e. Narrow upper and lower jaws

    f. Advance upper and lower jaws

    g. Early or late loss of baby teeth

h. Missing adult teeth

i. Difficulty with speech and chewing

j. Joint problems

DO I HAVE TO SEE ORTHODONTISTS FOR BRACES OR INVISALIGN®? MY DENTIST SAYS THEY CAN DO BRACES AND INVISALIGN® FOR ME.

A dentist is similar to your family doctor. Dentists are great for checkups, filling cavities, cleaning your teeth, and restoring your teeth with crowns and dentures. An orthodontist is a specialist who is a dentist and receives an additional 2-3 more years of education at an accredited orthodontic residency program. An orthodontist is an EXPERT in skeletal and dental growth and development, straightening your teeth and fixing a variety of your bite problems.

Some dentists may obtain additional weekends or short periods of orthodontic continuing education course training, and attempt to treat patients with braces or Invisalign® in their practices.

An orthodontist typically treats 200 to 600 patients with braces or Invisalign® per year; a dentist may treat less than 20 patients with braces or Invisalign® a year. As a comparison, when you need heart surgery, do you want your family doctor or a heart surgeon to operate on your heart?

Only orthodontists are accepted as members of the American Association of Orthodontists (AAO). Selecting an orthodontist who is the member of the AAO assures you that you are selecting an orthodontist. If you are not sure whether your dentists who are offering braces or Invisalign® to you are orthodontists, simply ask if they have completed the 2 to 3 year orthodontic residency training. You can also visit: www.braces.org to find an orthodontist in your zip code area.

ARE THERE DIFFERENCES AMONG ORTHODONTISTS?

As an orthodontist and a mom myself, I came up with a simple formula for you to choose your orthodontist for you and your family:

A chosen orthodontist = Dr. and staff clinical skill + Dr. personality + Office customer service

Orthodontics is a combination of art and science! Lots of patients consider all orthodontists to be the same! But . . .

...NOT ALL ORTHODONTISTS ARE THE SAME!

I will offer a checklist for you to choose the right orthodontist for you and your family:

#1. Do you take out my teeth?

Some orthodontists may prefer to extract your teeth, and some may prefer not to extract your teeth. I have had some patients come to me and mention that I am their third "stop", since the prior two orthodontists offered different opinions that confused them a lot. One orthodontist told them extraction was needed, and the second claimed no extraction was needed.

Remember, an orthodontist is an artist and a scientist! Art is not purely scientific! Therefore, different orthodontists will have different opinions about how your smile, teeth, lips, chin and face will look.

A good orthodontist will analyze the pros and cons of extraction vs non-extraction, and will make a final decision together with the patients. After all, it is your smile and face that you have to live with for the rest of your life. Make sure you are comfortable with the treatment decision!

#2. What kind of appliances do you use?

We orthodontists use different tools to straighten your teeth. The traditional braces offer metal and clear brackets. Patients will also have Invisalign® and lingual braces as choices, too.

Some orthodontists will claim they offer a certain "brand" of brackets which are superior to other brands. **To me, I think that is just a marketing gimmick and completely foolish!** There are hundreds of different bracket brands in the world. Orthodontists may have their preferences and claim some are better than others. To be honest with you, I have used lots of different brands of brackets, and they are almost equally good. Due to the good technology nowadays, most of the brackets on the markets can all deliver superior results. Again, it is a doctor's preference. To give you some insider information, I have heard that there are some orthodontists who use "recycled brackets" to lower the cost. The owner of the recycled company is actually a reputable professor. I know "recycle" does not sound good in your mouth, and though there are companies offering decent finished products, I prefer not to use them.

#3. Advanced training

Some orthodontists may have advanced training in joint problems, cleft palates/lips, surgical orthodontics, miniscrew anchorages, or Wilcodontics (A periodontal procedure which can finish your braces in 6-9 months). I think ninety percent of our patients fall in easy-to-moderate cases. However, there will be about ten percent of our patients whose treatment is genuinely challenging, and knowledgeable orthodontists do make big differences.

Another example is about second molars, or your twelve year molars. Lots of orthodontists nowadays do not treat second molars, and most patients will not know the difference. In my offices, we consider straightening second molars to be part of the end result we insist on delivering to our patients.

#4. Do you see patients on time? What is the percentage of treatments that are finished on time?

As a mother of two myself, I know how busy a mom and children can be with family, school, and work. Your precious time is important and should be cherished! A good orthodontic office will strive to see and finish patient treatment on time. In our office, we consider that we are seeing patients late if they have to wait for more than 3 minutes. Also, a good orthodontist should finish a patient's treatment on time at least 98 % of the time.

#5. How do I pay for my treatment?

Most orthodontic offices will work with you to customize a financial payment plan for you and your family. Some offices may require higher down payments to start the treatment, and some offices may be willing to start patients with lower down payments.

If you cannot come up with the minimal down payment to start treatment, look into third party financing, such as Springstone or Carecredit. These plans typically require decent credit history.

#6. Is there any charge for emergency visits?

Frankly, patients rarely undergo a "true emergency" situation during orthodontic treatment. Most "emergency" situations are comprised of loose bands or brackets, and pokey wires. Most offices will repair the appliances with no additional charges. However, most offices will charge an additional repair fee if patients have more excessive appliance breakage issues than normal.

Some visits will also have additional fees applied, such as lost Invisalign® trays and retainers – which I do consider an "emergency".

#7. How much does it cost? What is included in my treatment fee?

This is one of the most concerned questions a patient or parents will ask. I think the cost is important, but should not be the main determining factor in choosing your orthodontist. Remember, you are not only selecting a doctor to straighten your teeth, you are also selecting an "artist" who you will periodically see every couple of months to enhance your smile and personal experience.

There are lots of tangible factors you can judge, such as the type of appliances used, how long the treatment will be, how many sets of retainers, and if any teeth need to be removed.

The non-measurable factors may be the treatment finish-on-time rate, the overall treatment result, patient experience and satisfaction. You will be seeing the orthodontist for the next two to three years every couple of months. You better make sure that this is the office and doctors you want to visit, not just the "cheapest."

#8. Are the orthodontic offices privately owned or corporately owned?

I own my orthodontic offices, and all my colleagues and team members treat our patients like their family members. I know some orthodontists and dentists will not like what I am about to say. Frankly, I have to tell you that the "privately owned" orthodontic offices are more willing to go the "extra mile" for their patients as compared to the "corporately owned" ones, and offer a higher standard of patient care and customer service as well. The bottom line is to find an office that will treat you like a VIP, instead of just another patient who gets braces from them.

#9. Do you feel comfortable with the office atmosphere? Do you feel special and get a good first impression on the first visit?

Again, trust your instincts. Your orthodontist and staff should try their best to provide you with the most extraordinary experience and results, not just as another patient starting with braces. Your orthodontist should take excellent care of you from the initial consultation visit till the day you finish your treatment. Some orthodontic offices may cost less, but they may not go the "extra mile" for you during and after treatment.

#10. Are your orthodontic assistants registered dental assistants?

You will find that most of your orthodontic adjustment procedures will be executed by orthodontic assistants under the supervision of your orthodontist. Therefore, it is imperative to have high quality orthodontic assistants work on you and your family.

In certain states, it is mandatory that dental assistants go to additional dental assistant school training for several months to a year, and then pass the dental board exam to be qualified as an "RDA", Registered Dental Assistant.

There are also lots of states which do not require assistants to go through additional dental assistant school training to be an orthodontist assistant. Lots of orthodontists will hire their orthodontist assistants from Craigslist, neighbors or churches, and train them as apprentices.

In our offices, we only hire high-quality, experienced and certified dental assistants.

#11. Does your orthodontist offer a life-time warranty?

Believe or not, my offices do. During my years of practice, I encountered numerous patients who needed to get braces again, and I felt horrible and sorry about it! Trust me! I would rather have my patients have beautiful smiles for a lifetime, instead of charging them to have braces again. Therefore, we decided to offer a lifetime warranty for our patients, which is like life insurance to protect you for rest of your life! Isn't that a cool thing?

CHAPTER 2

TOP TEN REASONS YOU NEED BRACES

Believe it or not! We have surveyed thousands of our patients. Here are the top ten reasons why people are getting orthodontic treatment:

1. My smile does not look right! I want my smile to look perfect!

2. I am always embarrassed to smile for pictures.

3. I need to take pictures with a perfect smile for my graduation.

4. I need to take pictures with a perfect smile for my wedding.

5. I have a bad bite!

6. I have an "overbite".

7. I can't floss and brush my teeth well. They are too crooked!

8. My dentist said I need braces.

9. I have a narrow smile! I want to feel good about myself and my looks!

10. My kids are teased at school.

You will see that the number one reason people undergo orthodontic treatment is the desire **to look good and be confident**. A human's subconscious desire is to be praised, envied, noticed and needed. Having a perfect, white smile definitely is a symbol of youth and attraction, not just for ladies, but for gentlemen, too! Hey guys, do not tell me you don't care to look or feel good!

Can you recall the time in between losing your upper baby front teeth and waiting for your adult teeth to come out? I remember I was teased by my friends because I looked "funny", and I refused to smile until a couple years later. It was a traumatizing experience for me, and I can still recall the memory of my seven-year-old self being teased. Most patients will not notice how misaligned their bites are, but they will notice how bad their teeth look. Also, crooked teeth have been linked to the images of "lower social status" and "indifference"!

Other important reasons to have orthodontic treatment are for health and comfort. Crooked teeth have been linked to the potential development of periodontal disease and cavities, since it is challenging to brush and floss crooked teeth thoroughly. Misaligned bites are also linked to traumatized gums, severe wear of teeth, headaches, joint problems, snoring, and sinus problems.

We all want the best for our children and family. Having the orthodontic treatment with the right orthodontist will be your best and most inexpensive investment for a lifetime!

Be healthy, confident and fabulous!

CHAPTER 3

WHEN IS THE BEST TIME TO START ORTHODONTIC TREATMENT?

WHAT IS A GOOD AGE TO START BRACES?

The American Association of Orthodontics recommends all children should be seen by orthodontists **NO LATER THAN the AGE of 7!** Yes! Please call your orthodontist now if your children are older than 7 years old but have not seen orthodontists. I am not trying to scare you, but some parents may regret not doing so down the road.

In my practices, there are less than 5% of my patients who really need to start treatment before age of 10. Most children will not start braces till the age of 10-11. Girls typically can start braces earlier at the age of 10, since girls' growth and development are earlier than boys'. We often see some boys who do not start braces till an age of 13-14 due to their late growth and development.

Almost all orthodontists offer complimentary consultations for children's first consultations and typically continue to monitor them periodically – every 6-12 months – until they are ready for braces. Why not take great advantage of this opportunity for the experts to closely monitor your children's growth and development? It is almost literally free!

As I mentioned earlier, there are less than 5% of our children who really need to have some sort of orthodontic treatment prior to age of 10. Some orthodontists call it "phase I", and some call it "limited early treatment". Patients may need braces again at the age of 11-13, called "phase II". Here is a list of some of the definite criteria why we orthodontists can't wait until a later age to treat your children:

- Cross bite for back teeth

- Cross bite for front teeth (underbite)

- Limited cross bite of front teeth causing gum recession of lower front teeth

- Protrusive front teeth which may be easily traumatized from accidents

- Impacted adult teeth

- Early loss of baby teeth

- Thumb sucking habits with front teeth open bite

- Children are teased at school due to crooked or funny-looking teeth

- Children may have a speech problem due to the bite

- Cleft lips and palate

Unfortunately, these patients who need "phase I" at an early stage may still need full braces (phase II) again at a later age. This two-phase treatment always carries a higher cost of treatment fees for the parents and longer treatment time for the children. Luckily, not too many children require early treatment.

Other than the above problems I mentioned above that must be treated immediately, most of our children can start braces about age 11. Some orthodontists will preach early treatment to avoid future extraction or jaw surgery in the future. However, well-designed research has shown that early treatment will not prevent future extraction or jaw surgery. Most of the problems can be treated with one-time braces when our children are age 11-13, and it delivers almost identical results with children who have braces twice.

Some parents may be very confused why certain orthodontists want to do something now and some ask you to wait? Well, it all depends on your orthodontist's philosophy and how comfortable you feel about your children's teeth and looks. It won't hurt to improve our children's appearance and confidence at their young age if orthodontic treatment is affordable.

CAN ADULTS HAVE BRACES, TOO?
WILL ADULT'S TEETH MOVE SLOWER THAN KIDS?

Can you believe that I did not get braces till I was twenty-six years old? I would not regret it to do it again! Adult can absolutely have orthodontic treatment! Some adult patients never had a chance to have braces at an earlier age (I am one of them), or they had braces before, but the teeth are crooked again due to not wearing retainers.

Will adult's teeth move slower than kids'? Research showed that adults may take a little bit longer for teeth to start moving. Once adult's teeth start to move, the speed is actually the same as that of kids. The most challenging aspects for adult patients are not the speed. Adult patients tend to have missing teeth, joint discomfort, crowned teeth and existing periodontal problems. These conditions usually complicate the orthodontic treatment results and slow down the tooth movement.

I am a great advocate of adults having orthodontic treatment. Our adult patients are so lucky nowadays to have several invisible choices, such as Invisalign®, clear and lingual braces, to achieve lifetime fabulous smiles

CHAPTER 4

TREATMENT OPTIONS FOR ORTHODONTIC TREATMENT

We orthodontists use many appliances to straighten your teeth, improve your jaw alignment, improve your look, and speed up your treatment. There are hundreds of orthodontic appliances on the market, and here are the most common ones you will hear:

For younger ages:
- Palatal expander
- Space maintainer
- Functional appliances
- Headgear and Chin cup
- Thumb sucking crib

For teen and adult ages:
- Metal braces
- Clear braces
- Invisalign® and Invisalign Teen®
- Lingual braces

For people who want to speed up treatment time:
- Wilcodontics
- Acceledent
- Suresmile

WHAT IS AN EXPANDER? WILL I AVOID EXTRACTION IF I USE EXPANDERS?

Expanders are two-pieced acrylic or metal plates connected with a screw in the middle. For the upper arch, palatal expanders are glued at the roof of your palate to widen your arch in younger patients less than 15-17 years old. I do not use expanders in the lower arch since the result is very limited due to the anatomical restriction of the lower arch. Expanders are used in patients with narrower upper arches and wider lower arches, called a crossbite. After the expander is placed and glued in the mouth, the patient is instructed to use a "key" to activate the expander one to two times a day. After orthodontists achieve the desired amount of expansion, expanders will be "secured" and stay in the mouth for a few more months to ensure the widened arch stays in the same place and does not "shrink back".

Once the expander is "activated" and the arch starts getting wider, most patients will encounter a "pressure" feeling around the face, talk funny, and drool sometimes. The "pressure" sensation usually disappears in the next couple of hours after "activation." Most patients will get used to it and not feel "funny" or drool after three days. Brushing is more challenging when you have an expander. Believe me, you need to brush your teeth AND the expander while it stays in your mouth.

It is common for an expander to dislodge from one of your teeth, especially when patients have significant expansion. We advise that you try to place the expander back in your mouth and call the office immediately for repair. It is easy to glue an expander back into your mouth if you keep it in the mouth. Once it is out of the mouth completely, it is very challenging to glue the expander back and we may need to give you a new expander.

Can we avoid extraction by expanding the arch only? The answer is yes for the upper teeth, but no for the lower teeth. The upper arch's anatomy has a suture in the middle of the palate, which has soft cartilage and can be elastically stretched by the palatal expander in younger ages (less than 15-17 years old). If the suture in the palate has fused, (typically when older than 15-17 years old), then it will be very hard to widen the suture and palate, rather than "tip" all the upper teeth outward.

The problem in using an expander in the lower arch is that we do not have a suture in the middle of the mandible to expand. Lots of times we only "tip" or "flare" the teeth out of the supporting bone, but not by moving or expanding the bone. The long term result is unstable and unpredictable, and extraction is the best solution if patient has too much crowding.

WHAT IS A SPACE MAINTAINER?

Space maintainers are the appliances customized by your orthodontist or pedodontist to "keep or maintain" the space required for adult tooth eruption after losing baby teeth too early due to extraction by decay. If the space is not maintained properly after losing the baby teeth, the other teeth may shift to the open space and close the space needed for the adult teeth to come out. It will cause severe problems for upcoming adult teeth, such as impacted adult teeth or a wrong bite.

There are two types of space maintainers, removable and fixed. Removable space maintainers are made of acrylic and with artificial teeth added to hold the space for unerupted adult teeth. Patients can take it out anytime. Fixed space maintainers are glued into your month, and patients need to avoid chewy or sticky food that can dislodge the appliances. All space maintainers need to be closely monitored by your orthodontist periodically to ensure that they are not interfering with any adult teeth eruption. Patients will be instructed to stop wearing the space maintainers when ready for orthodontic treatment.

WHAT IS A FUNCTIONAL APPLIANCE?

Functional appliances are more popular in the European countries than in the United States. They are designed to move both the teeth and the jaws, especially the lower jaws, and mold your muscle, cheeks and tongue. They are particularly used during children's younger ages, prior to fixed brace treatment to promote lower jaw development. There are so many functional appliances on the market, such as Herbst appliances, Twin blocks, Myra... you name it. The treatment time is usually 9 to 12 months and most patients will need braces.

Headgear and chin cup:

Headgear is often used to fix problems for people who have protrusive front teeth (excessive overjet). It is supported by the "head" and connected to the upper molars to restrict the upper jaw and promote lower jaw growth. Most patients will wear braces at the same time to help "push" the upper front teeth backward. The main difference between a Herbst functional appliance and headgear is that a Herbst appliance is glued to your teeth, while headgear is removable. Headgear needs to be worn in the mouth around 16 hours a day in order to see desirable results. Headgear should not be worn while playing sports or while eating.

A chin cup is another add-on treatment for growing patients who have a prominent lower jaw, which is what we call an underbite. The chin cup's purpose is to apply pressure on the temporomandibular joint to inhibit or redirect lower jaw growth. It is more commonly used by Asian than Caucasian or Hispanic patients.

Thumb sucking stopping appliances:

What is the big deal about our children sucking their thumbs or using a pacifier on a daily basis? It is no big deal before children have their anterior adult teeth erupt. It will be a BIG deal when children start having adult teeth but still suck their thumb. The common side effects of thumb sucking at an older age include a narrow upper arch, flared out upper front teeth and reclined lower front teeth, and a mostly anterior open bite.

There are several approaches to stop thumb sucking behavior. I usually explain to the children, not the parents, how bad they are going to look if they do not stop sucking their thumb. We encourage parents and children to work as a team to seriously stop this detrimental habit by closely monitoring their progress, and rewarding them accordingly every three months. If the habits cannot be stopped, further thumb sucking appliances will be considered.

WHY DO PEOPLE STILL WEAR METAL BRACES?

Most patients hesitate to wear braces due to the look of metal braces. The reason we orthodontists still use metal braces is because they produce less friction than ceramic braces, less chances to chip off, and tend to move teeth faster. Ironically, I myself had braces twice in my twenties. I wore clear braces the first time, and metal braces the second time for one year right after I finished my original treatment, since I wanted to emphasize treatment efficiency more than my appearance of wearing braces.

I always tell my patients to **SHOW OFF** your metal braces, instead of hiding them. Why? Wearing braces is the symbol of "I am taking care of myself to have a lifetime, fabulous smile; my parents care about taking care of me." Why not "dress up" your metal braces to be part of your personal statement and distinguish your characters. You can change your braces color to match the colors of your favorite sport teams or school. You can be creative in wearing different patterns on your braces. You can match your colors according to the holidays, such as Halloween, Christmas, St. Patrick's Day, or Valentine's Day.

Wearing braces can be fun and stylish!

WHAT ARE CLEAR BRACES?

The majority of clear braces are ceramic, and they will give you the "metal-free" look while straightening your smile. Our adult patients love it! Some of our young teenagers, such as ballerina and drama performers, prefer braces treatment with the almost invisible look of ceramic braces.

I myself love the look of ceramic braces, too. From the treatment efficiency point of view, I recommend all my patients to have upper clear braces, but not for all of the lower arches. There are two scenarios in which I prefer not to have clear braces in the lower arch: Patients with severe lower anterior crowding and deep overbite. Clear braces tend to decrowd the crooked teeth slower when the teeth are extremely crowded. Clear braces also tend to wear off upper front teeth due to the stiffer material – especially for deepbite patients.

INVISALIGN®: TRUTH VS MYTH

Invisalign® has been around the market for more than 20 years. I still remember when it first appeared in one of TIME magazine's issues talking about how orthodontists will be obsolete due to the innovation of Invisalign®. Invisalign® is truly an amazing and invisible tool to straighten your smile without wearing braces at all.

How does Invisalign® work? Your orthodontist will take impressions or scan your tooth images to Align Technology. Upon receiving the images of your teeth, Align Technology will use 3D software to simulate tooth movement to the final best positions. Orthodontists will predict, plan, communicate and instruct Align Technology on the requirements for the "prescription" to correct your crooked teeth and bite. Upon approval by your orthodontist, Align Technology will fabricate a series of customized trays ready for you to wear.

Myth #1: All patients are eligible for Invisalign®.
Truth: Invisalign® technology has been improving to treat more complicated cases nowadays. However, there still will be lots of more complicated treatments that can't be accomplished efficiently and effectively by Invisalign® treatment, such as severe bite problems and extraction cases.

Myth #2: Invisalign® moves teeth faster than braces.
Truth: Invisalign® moves the teeth at the same speed as braces. Invisalign® and braces are just different tools to

apply pressure to your teeth and create tooth movement. Your teeth have no idea whether this comes from the plastic tray or metal wires.

Myth #3: Invisalign® treatment is shorter than braces.

Truth: As I mentioned, Invisalign® moves your teeth at the same rate as braces. Orthodontists tend to offer Invisalign® for relatively simple to moderate cases, which results in the false impression that Invisalign® has a shorter treatment time.

Myth #4: All dentists can provide Invisalign® treatment.

Truth: When Invisalign® was first launched, it could only be distributed strictly to orthodontists. The general dentists saw the potential consumer demand and financial rewards, and took legal action to request the Invisalign® company to distribute the products to "all dental professionals", and not limited to "orthodontists" only. Thereafter, Invisalign® can be purchased at either a dentist's or an orthodontist's offices.

If I offer you an airplane and give you a two-day crash course, will you hop on it, and feel confident flying to Europe? Or would you feel more confident having a pilot flying your plane who has gone through two to three years of intensive training for flying the plane? Having an airplane does not warrant you the comprehensive knowledge about how to fly. This analogy applies to Invisalign® treatment as well.

Myth #5: Invisalign® does not hurt as much as braces.

Truth: You will feel the same amount of pressure when your teeth start to move, whether it is by Invisalign® or braces. Your teeth can not differentiate between Invisalign® or braces moving your teeth.

Myth #6: Invisalign® is more expensive than braces.

Truth: It depends on the orthodontic office. It is true that Invisalign® has a higher cost of lab fees payable to Align Technology. Some orthodontic offices do charge more for Invisalign® due to the extra lab cost. However, the lab expenses are somehow compensated by less chair time patients spend in the office with less office and emergency visits. Therefore, we do not charge differently for Invisalign® and braces in our offices.

Invisalign® does offer great benefits:

✓ - Invisible look

✓ - No food restrictions: You can enjoy all your favorite food and not worry about breaking the appliances

✓ - Non-restricted life style: Your social life is not affected due to the invisible look and no food restriction

✓ - Fewer office and emergency visits to your orthodontist offices

✓ - Better oral hygiene

LINGUAL BRACES

Lingual braces, also a form of invisible braces, are brackets that are placed on the inside surfaces of your teeth, toward your tongue. If you literally ask for "invisible" braces, lingual braces should be the ultimate solution for you.

Unlike Invisalign®, which treats simple to moderate cases more efficiently, lingual braces can treat far more difficult cases. Lingual braces can be challenging for patients initially. Can you imagine your tongue having less space due to the thickness of lingual braces, and constantly being irritated by the braces? Most patients will have ulcers around the tongue and feel difficulty in talking. Luckily, most patients report getting used to lingual braces about two weeks later. Keeping your teeth clean while having lingual braces can be another issue, since lots of patients do not brush their inner-surface teeth, not to mention brushing lingual braces.

Due to the three-dimensional technology, lingual braces can be customized to treat patients' crooked teeth precisely and effectively. However, lingual braces may not be for everyone! First, I don't recommend lingual braces for patients who have an existing periodontal condition or poor oral hygiene, since lingual braces may aggravate the periodontal health more due to the nature of the braces' location. Second, lingual braces will not stay on the teeth if a patient has very small crowns. Third, lingual braces are more costly relative to traditional braces and lnvisalign. There will be lab fees involved to customize lingual braces. Doctor and staff chair time with lingual braces patients will be more, since they have to work on the patient's inner surfaces of the teeth. Last, you may not be a candidate for lingual braces if you are very "sensitive to new things" and have a low pain tolerance.

ARE THERE ANY WAYS TO "SPEED UP" MY ORTHODONTIC TREATMENT?

Lots of patients are discouraged from starting orthodontic treatment due to the long treatment time. Especially for adults, we can't imagine our busy daily life with the fact and "look" of braces! I hear you, since I mentioned that I had my braces TWICE in my twenties during my orthodontic residency at the University of Illinois at Chicago.

Yes, there are several conjunctive procedures and devices in the market that bring us hope to decrease orthodontic treatment time:

Wilcodontics (AOO™)

Wilcodontics is named after the brothers Dr. Thomas and William Wilco. One of the brothers is a periodontist, and the other is an orthodontist. The Wilcodontic procedure is a surgical procedure performed by periodontists to increase the bone turnover rate, thus decreasing the treatment time by 3 to 4 times over conventional orthodontics. This procedure is also known as Accelerated Osteogenic Orthodontics™ (AOO™).

I was an actual patient of AOO™ when I had my braces the second time during my orthodontic residency. I was eager to finish my orthodontic treatment in the shortest period of time, because it was my second time wearing braces. I happened to have a periodontist boyfriend, who is my dear husband now, and he was willing to try it on me. We went to Erie, Pennsylvania to get certified together, and I was his first AOO™ patient. The procedure was easy but time consuming! It took him about three hours to complete the procedure. My braces were finished in one year, despite an original estimated treatment time of eighteen to twenty months.

The great news is that AOO™ really works and can speed up your orthodontic treatment to less than a year. The long-term follow up shows stable bone healing with no additional side effects. The only downside is the cost. Since it is a meticulous, time-consuming and technique-sensitive procedure for the periodontist, it isn't cheap! You are looking at double your total cost for orthodontic treatment with the additional surgery fee. For example, you will spend an additional $5000 on the AOO™ procedure, if your orthodontic treatment fee is $5000.

Acceledent ™

There is a new orthodontic device called Acceledent™. It is a simple at-home mouthpiece device designed to move your teeth up to 50% faster for orthodontic treatment with 20 minutes daily use. It uses SoftPulse technology, which accelerates the bone remodeling process around your teeth. Acceledent™ also decreases the discomfort associated with orthodontic treatment clinically. It can be used with both patients wearing braces and Invisalign®. Ask your orthodontist to purchase Acceledent™, which will cost you about $750-$1000 per piece. Unlike AOO™ requiring a surgical procedure and higher cost, Acceledent™ is less invasive and more cost friendly. However, it requires faithful application of 20 minutes a day by patients at home for the whole length of orthodontic treatment. I wonder how many well-disciplined adult and teenager patients we will have nowadays?

Suresmile™

Suresmile™ is a computer-assisted orthodontic technology to help orthodontists and patients shorten the treatment time by 40% on average. Your orthodontist will start your braces to resolve crowding, close space, and reduce overjet and overbite for the initial to middle two-thirds of your treatment. The last one-third of your treatment time will be working on "finishing and detailing" your bite, your tooth final position, and ideal parallelism of your roots in the bone.

For the last one-third of your orthodontic treatment time, it typically takes up to eight to ten months, which varies by the skill of your orthodontist. The orthodontist will use pliers to bend archwires to move your teeth and roots in small increments. Sometimes it is time consuming and involves human error. With Suresmile™ technology, a three-dimensional scan was taken and sent to Suresmile™. The orthodontist will simulate what the final position of your teeth and roots will be and approve the treatment plan. In the same way Invisalign® fabricates a series of trays to correct teeth, Suresmile™ uses "robot- technology" to customize a series of arch wires to finalize a patient's final stage of treatment. With the elimination of human error and the "guessing" part of arch-wire adjustment, Suresmile™ can decrease the treatment time by up to 40%. For a 24-month treatment time, we are talking about finishing in 15 months.

Of course, patients will have to invest more treatment fees on this high end technology. If you want a faster and more predictable treatment result, and are not sensitive about treatment cost, then Suresmile™ is the way to go!

CHAPTER 5

WHY DO I NEED TEETH REMOVED FOR MY ORTHODONTIC TREATMENT?

There is a very interesting myth and misunderstanding about why orthodontists recommend removal of teeth for orthodontic treatment. Some patients are afraid that the remaining teeth are going to have "problems" down the road; some dentists even claim that removing teeth will "destroy" the face; some even believe that you absolutely can't take ANY TOOTH out of the mouth because they are part of your body.

The debate to extract or not has been an ongoing battle in the orthodontist world since the early twentieth century. For some cases on the borderline of extraction or not, most orthodontists nowadays will attempt to treat patients without taking the tooth out first, and then recommend extraction only when necessary. For some cases, extraction will be necessary in order to achieve a functional, esthetically-pleasing result. Lots of patients, even dentists, have misconceptions about "crowding," and believe that this is the only reason to remove teeth. Here are some consensuses about when to extract teeth for orthodontic treatment:

1. Teeth are way too crowded.

This is the obvious reason for removing teeth, and most patients or parents can understand easily without my persuasion. As I often mentioned, "You need to kick out some of the residents if you only have a small house. It will overcrowd the small house, and somebody needs to go."

2. Teeth are not too crowded, but the front teeth are sticking out and push the lips out.

The patient looks like they are holding a golf ball inside of the mouth. If you see these people from the side, you will easily see the top and bottom front teeth are flaring outward toward the lips. Most of these patients will have a hard time closing their lips in a relaxing way. Their face just looks mad and not relaxed. By extracting some premolar teeth in the back, it will move the flaring front teeth backward and retract the lips back. The end result is that patients can close their mouth easily and the face will look younger and more pleasant.

3. Patients desire to have a "straighter" profile, meaning a taller nose, a more prominent chin, and balanced lips.

Have you seen the Doctor 90210 show about the nose job and chin augmentation? People desire to have a taller nose and a more prominent chin. It just looks prettier! Do you know wearing braces only can give you the same "plastic surgery" result without going through painful scalpels? Using the same concept as #2, we can make over your look to achieve a taller nose and a better chin just by taking out some premolar teeth, and by moving the front teeth and lips way back.

4. The patient looks like "Austin Powers" with goofy protrusive top front teeth, and can barely keep the mouth closed.

The "Austin Powers" bite is what most patients refer to as, "I have an overbite." The top front teeth are sticking out so much that it gives patients a goofy look. Sadly, lots of kids, even adults, are teased because of this goofy look. Some easy cases can be easily treated without taking out teeth at a younger age. However, some cases will require removal of top premolars to push the upper front teeth back.

5. Patients have an underbite with lower teeth on top of upper teeth, and no jaw surgery is needed.

An underbite is what we refer to as a "bulldog bite" or an "anterior crossbite". It means that the lower anterior teeth are on top or ahead of the upper anterior teeth. By removing the lower premolars, it creates the space in the back to move the lower anterior teeth backwards.

6. Patients have some missing teeth, and we will have to extract additional teeth in order to match the bite.

For example, when patients are missing a couple lower teeth, we will have to remove a couple of the upper teeth to "match" the number of upper and lower teeth for the bite to fit together.

CHAPTER 6

DO I NEED TO REMOVE MY WISDOM TEETH?

Lots of patients ask me if they should remove their wisdom teeth. If yes, will it be before or after braces? Can the wisdom teeth be removed during the braces treatment?

Why do we call third molars "wisdom teeth?"

The name of "wisdom teeth," or third molars, derives from the fact that they usually appear in your mouth between the ages of 17 and 25, which is coincidentally the age that humans mature and develop their "wisdom." Wisdom teeth, if present, are the last teeth to develop and erupt. Most patients have missing, partially erupted, or completely impacted, wisdom teeth.

WHEN CAN I KEEP MY WISDOM TEETH?

You may keep your wisdom teeth if they are:

a. Completely erupted and have functional contacts against the opposing teeth on the opposite arch (give you more surfaces to chew).

b. No signs of cavity, pain and gum disease.

c. Easy to access for cleaning.

d. Checked annually with x-rays and follow ups by your dentist to ensure no pathological changes.

WHEN DO I HAVE TO REMOVE MY WISDOM TEETH?

In fact, 90% of our population has at least one wisdom tooth which does not fully grow into the mouth, thus, called an impacted wisdom tooth.

In general, wisdom teeth will need to be removed if they are:

    a. Constantly having issues with swelling, infection and/or giving you discomfort.

    b. Having gum disease and non-restorable cavities.

    c. Having cysts, tumors, or other pathologic changes.

    d. Causing damages or cavities to neighboring teeth.

    e. Having no functional contacts to bite against the opposing teeth.

SHOULD I REMOVE MY WISDOM TEETH BEFORE, DURING OR AFTER BRACES?

It is not mandatory to extract your wisdom teeth prior to braces, unless you have encountered problems with wisdom tooth eruption. There are very few occasions we orthodontists ask our patients to remove wisdom teeth to assist with braces treatment.

If wisdom teeth start to erupt during orthodontic treatment and they are giving you discomfort, they can be removed during the orthodontic treatment.

Most patients remove their wisdom teeth after completion of braces. Some oral surgeons believe it is better to remove wisdom teeth before the roots complete formation, since younger adults are more likely to recover faster with less complications from surgery than elderly adults.

WILL WISDOM TEETH MAKE MY TEETH CROOKED AFTER BRACES?

This is the most common question asked by my patients and parents. It is a common misconception that wisdom teeth will make your teeth crooked again!

The general consensus is that wisdom teeth WILL NOT make your teeth crooked again after braces as long as you WEAR YOUR RETAINERS! Not wearing retainers will cost you crooked teeth again, not your wisdom teeth!

CHAPTER 7

ORTHODONTIC FINANCE

1. How much do braces cost?

As a mother of two, I think my children's lifetime-lasting, healthy, pretty smiles and confidence are "priceless". As an orthodontic patient myself, I can't imagine myself having crooked teeth for even one second. To me, having crooked teeth is worse than having wrinkles on my forehead. In general, I would say braces typically range from $4000 to $8000 for a full case treatment.

I have some patients who consulted with three orthodontists and asked me why the treatment fee ranges significantly among offices. As I mentioned in my earlier chapter, not all orthodontists are the same. Please refer to the Chapter "How to Choose the Right Orthodontist." When you buy a dream house for you and your family, you will have an ideal picture in your mind about what you will be looking for in your dream house. You may consider location to be the number one concern: that it needs to be close to your work for example. You may consider certain locations to be desirable, but it may be far from where you work. You may want to buy the most plain and basic house at a dirt cheap price, and plan to spend tons of time and money to improve the condition. You may also choose to buy the most impressive mansion which may be pricier, but you know that it has everything to fit your needs and will be your dream house.

The same concept applies to the cost of orthodontic treatment. Orthodontic treatment is not just about gluing a set of brackets or delivering a set of Invisalign® trays to your teeth. Orthodontic treatment is not just about changing wires and moving your teeth. A good orthodontist invests lots of money on constantly bettering his or her clinical skills and efficiency. For example, the offices will have frequent customer service and continuing education training for their staff, or the orthodontist may invest money to enhance the patient experience and satisfaction throughout the treatment. They may hire more experienced certified orthodontic assistants to take care of their patients. It all costs more than just "straighten my crooked teeth!" There can be extra sweat and efforts, and of course, the cost beyond the theme.

You can have your children spend a whole day playing in the community park, which will cost you nothing. You can also drive or fly hours to spend a whole day at Disneyland, which will cost you more, but the experience is far more memorable than "basic".

2. How do I pay for my braces?

a. Payment plans

Most orthodontic offices offer a 0% interest payment plan to finance your treatment fee with affordable monthly installments spread out during your treatment time. Unlike loaning money from your traditional bank, you literally loan the treatment fee from your orthodontist without paying an interest charge. Who said there is no free lunch in the world?

b. Pay-in-full

Most orthodontic offices love to offer you a pay-in-full discount if you can make a onetime payment.

c. Third party financing

There are hundreds of vendors out there who are willing to finance your orthodontic treatment should you have decent credit history. The major medical third party finance vendors are CareCredit and Lending Club. Lots of orthodontic offices are actually paying a 15-20% transaction fee for you if you are qualified. This is an excellent option to pay for your braces with no initial down payment and small monthly payments. Make sure you ask your orthodontic office about this option.

d. Flexible Spending Accounts
Please refer to p.53 – #5. How do I use Flexible Spending Accounts for my orthodontic treatment?

3. Tips to save cost for orthodontic treatment

a. Pay your fee in full.
Most orthodontic offices offer 5% to 10% discount for paid-in-full payment. It saves offices the administrative and labor fees to charge your bank or credit card monthly. Some of my patients' families get a small loan from "0% interest credit line" from the bank for one year. Some patients ask for help from their grandparents or relatives to get an advanced loan. I also have encountered patients that set up a "smile fund" and put money aside monthly to pay for braces or Invisalign® in full.

b. Sign up for your braces with your family members or friends.
Most orthodontists are happy to offer family bundle discounts or multiple-people discounts.

c. Make appointments during downtime.
Most orthodontists are slower during school hours, typically in the morning and before 2:00 in the afternoon. Ask your orthodontist for a break if you restrict your appointments to downtime.

d. Be a compliant patient and the best team player.
Some offices offer incentives if patients never miss appointments and have no loose appliances throughout the total treatment.

e. Use a Flexible Spending Account.

f. Take advantage of promotions.
Orthodontics are a small business after all. We may

occasionally run promotions to take some dollar amount off your treatment fee. Watch out for the special offers in the May or December seasons.

g. Ask for a student or military discount.
Depending on the philosophy of orthodontists, some will offer some sort of discounts or a couple hundred dollars off to help with self-paid students and to pay tribute to the military family.

4. How does orthodontic insurance work?

Most orthodontic insurances are "lifetime" benefit, not "yearly" benefit. Unlike your dental insurances which have a yearly maximum, orthodontic insurances only offer a one-time, lifetime benefit. For example, if your plan has a $1,000 dental and $1,000 orthodontic coverage, you will have $1,000 to spend every year on your dental work, but your insurance will only pay for your braces up to a total of $1,000 throughout your two-year orthodontic treatment. Most orthodontic insurances spread out the $1,000 for two years. The insurance company usually breaks down payments monthly or quarterly to your orthodontist. Should patients lose their orthodontic insurances during the middle of the treatment, they will not pay the full $1,000 benefit. The unpaid insurance balance will then be transferred to the patient's responsible portion.

Many patients may have two orthodontic insurances from both parents. It does not guarantee the full payments from both insurance plans. Some insurance plans have a "coordination of benefit" clause. Depending on which insurance is primary, some secondary insurances will pay minimal or even no payment toward your orthodontic treatment if the primary insurance pays more or equal to the secondary insurance benefit. Orthodontic insurances can be confusing! Make sure you understand your insurance plan or ask the insurance specialist at your orthodontist's to help you with the questions.

5. How do I use Flexible Spending Accounts for my orthodontic treatment?

Flexible Spending Accounts (FSA's) are a way to pay out-of-pockct (un-reimbursed) health care expenses, (Medical FSA) and dependent care expenses (Dependent Care FSA) on a PRE-TAX basis!

Orthodontic services are not provided in the same way as other types of health care are. Most of the time they are provided over a long period of time and will extend beyond a plan year. Orthodontic services tend to be hard to match up with the actual costs, and, as a result, the reimbursement process is different. Normally there are two ways to be reimbursed:

1. Entire cost of treatment- This method allows you to be reimbursed for the full amount of the Orthodontic contract. You can only do this if you paid the full contract amount during the plan year. To get reimbursed you must send in the following items:

    - Completed reimbursement request form.

    - Proof of payment for the entire contract, including start date and expected end date.

    - Proof of payment made during the applicable plan year in which you are requesting reimbursement.

2. Monthly approach- This method allows you to be reimbursed for the first round of treatment (usually called banding fees) and then monthly reimbursement after that. To get reimbursed for banding fees, you must submit:

    - Completed reimbursement request form.

    - Your treatment plan or itemized statement that includes the start date and the expected end date.

    - Proof of initial down payment.

After you submit the first reimbursement request, send in these items for monthly reimbursement:

- Completed reimbursement request form.

- An itemized statement or monthly coupons from the Orthodontist.

- Proof of the monthly payment.

CHAPTER 8

TAKING CARE OF YOUR BRACES

SECTION I.
HOW TO CLEAN MY BRACES? HOW TO AVOID A PERMANENT BRACKET-MARK ON MY TEETH?

We often hear horrible stories that wearing braces leaves your teeth with white, nasty spots and lots of cavities. The real answer to these stories is true and false. It is true that very few patients "create" white spots along the brackets and gum line after finishing orthodontic treatment. The braces themselves will NOT cause it. It is the lack of brushing and flossing (laziness and carelessness) that is the main culprit. Most people don't realize how easy it is to clean your braces and teeth during orthodontic treatment. Here are some main tips that I guarantee will prevent cavities while wearing braces:

1. Try to brush your teeth <u>right after eating</u>. If you don't have a toothbrush, rinse your mouth at least. If you don't have tooth paste, brush without it.

2. How many times should you brush your teeth? Right after eating and drinking. I know it is impossible! The most important time to brush and floss is before you go to bed. You absolutely CAN NOT skip this one.

3. There are two areas that are the most important to brush: along the junction of your gum and teeth, and also the area around the brackets. Make sure to brush your teeth

55

above the brackets and below the brackets. Also, gently message your gum area.

4. After brushing, always go to the mirror and check if there is still debris on your teeth. Stretch your cheeks to check your back teeth and lower front teeth. Most people only brush their upper front teeth well.

5. Electronic tooth brushes are very efficient and helpful. However, you can brush your teeth excellently without using electronic ones. The same concept applies to water picks and mouth rinse. Thorough brushing is the key, not the tools.

6. Nothing can replace flossing. You really need to use **superfloss** to assist in passing the floss though the wires every time you floss. It scrapes things between your teeth. Rule of thumb, <u>always floss before you go to sleep</u> if you cannot do this during the daytime.

7. Make sure you go to your family dentist every 3-6 months for routine cleanings and check-ups. We always encourage our patients to remove the archwires with us first before your cleaning appointments, since your dentist can access your teeth easier and clean more efficiently.

8. Replace your toothbrush when you see it wears out.

SECTION II.
WHAT FOOD CAN I AND CAN'T
I EAT WHILE WEARING BRACES?

I always tell my patients you basically can enjoy all kinds of your food during braces. It is <u>HOW</u> you eat your food, not what you eat. The #1 golden rule is to *cut your food into small pieces before any food enters your mouth.* You will have to use a knife or scissors to cut your food, <u>not your teeth</u>. The #2 golden rule is to avoid anything hard, chunky, chewy, sticky and high in sugar content. The hard, chewy food can break brackets and archwires, and sticky food can pop the bands out. The #3 golden rule is take some over-the-counter painkillers for the first 3-5 days when you just get braces or a new adjustment.

1. Food that is friendly to braces:
   Soups, noodles, spaghetti, pasta, mac and cheese, eggs, healthy nutrient shakes and yogurt.

2. Food to try to avoid with braces:
   Hard: Ice cubes, popcorn, nuts, hard candies, corn on the cobs, pizza crust. When eating fresh fruits (apples, etc.) and hard raw vegetables (carrots, celeries, etc.), slice them thinly. Meat (ribs and chickens) should be off the bone and cut into small pieces. Chewing or biting on any hard object such as pencils, silverware, nails, and keys.

   Chewy: Gum, beef jerky, gummy bears.

   Sticky: Caramel, taffy apples, Starburst candies, Jolly Ranchers, and sticky rice.

   Food with high sugar content: Soda, milkshakes and ice cream (brush your teeth immediately).

SECTION III.
WHY DO I HAVE "BROKEN BRACKETS OR LOOSE BANDS" ALL THE TIME?

There are always certain patients who always have loose brackets/bands. When it happens, parents or patients always question us if the "glue" we use is not strong enough, or we may not glue the braces properly.

Parents and patients, listen, braces or bands WILL NOT come off themselves unless patients BITE THEM OFF. We orthodontists use the best glues to secure the braces strong enough to stay on your teeth during the treatment, but not too strong to damage your enamels while taking them off. We would love to use SUPERGLUES, of course, to make sure all the braces will definitely STAY on your teeth. However, can you imagine how superglue can take off all your tooth structures when we try to remove the brackets upon finishing your treatment?

There are several reasons to have "broken brackets":

1. Not cutting your food into small pieces. **RULE OF THUMB: CUT ALL FOOD INTO SMALL SLICES!** Please refer to Question #2. Again, be like ladies and gentleman while having braces in your mouth, use a knife (not your teeth) to cut everything into small pieces, no matter if it is hard or soft!

2. Patients have severe overbite, which usually causes breakage of lower braces. We orthodontists will typically use special tools, such as build-up bumps, bite-turbo, bite blocks, or bite pillows, to raise up your bite.

3. You have bad habits such as biting nails, chewing ice, pens and pencils.

4. Your bite has been changed due to the movement of your teeth and you now may be biting on the braces.

In our office, we run a "stress test" on our cemented brackets after placing brackets on the patients. We intentionally test and press the brackets HARD to see if the new-glued brackets will resist the sufficient strength. It shows our patients and parents that the braces stay very strong and are cemented properly.

SECTION IV.
WHAT TO DO WHEN I HAVE
LOOSE BANDS OR BRACKETS?

Luckily, there is truly NO EMERGENCY for orthodontic treatment, unless your arch wire pokes through your eye balls!

1. If you plan to be on vacation, make sure to bring some "wax" with you. Place wax at discomfort area for temporary relief until you are back from vacation. Most of the time you can wait to get loose braces repaired when you are back. If it is really bothering you, you can call a local orthodontist for assistance for an office visit fee.

2. Call your orthodontist right away. If you are due for an adjustment within a few days of the bracket becoming loose, your orthodontist may suggest that you to wait until your upcoming scheduled appointment. If your next appointment isn't for a few weeks, your orthodontist may give you an earlier appointment to repair your loose braces. Either way, **we orthodontists would want to be informed**, so we are able to prepare in advance for the extra time that is required to repair your loose appliances.

3. It is common for a loose bracket to "slide" along the wire. If there is no discomfort, leave it as it is and call your orthodontist. If the bracket is rubbing on the gum, place a piece of the orthodontic wax over the loose bracket area. If you don't have any wax, use a piece of sugar-free gum instead.

4. If you have a loose band (ring), try to push the band back to the tooth and call your orthodontist. Please avoid any sticky food, which will "pop" your bands out again.

5. If the brackets or bands come off, try to save them in Ziploc® bags and bring them to your orthodontist for repair.

Remember, when your braces become loose, the teeth involved are no longer moving. Having your braces become loose may set your treatment back by months - because the teeth will then need to "catch-up" to the other teeth around it. Sadly, I had a couple of patients that had loose brackets several days before getting braces off, which cost them a couple more months of delay for the braces to come off.

SECTION V.
WHAT TO DO WITH POKEY WIRES?

Honestly, the best way to avoid pokey wires is by prevention! I have to say that some of the orthodontic assistants do not always clip the back wire short enough at the adjustment visits (human errors). Make sure to always "feel" your mouth and make sure nothing is pokey or bothering you at the end of your adjustment visit. It typically prevents at least 60% of the pokey wire issues.

Pokey wires frequently occur when patients just get their braces on. The reason is that we orthodontists use initial "skinny and flexible wires" to level and straighten your crooked teeth. Therefore, the flexible wires may slide along, making one side of the wire longer and the other side of the wire shorter. The wires may even slip out of the back teeth's bracket slots. If the wire comes out of the tube, try to use tweezers to place the wire back in front of a mirror, or ask somebody do it for you. If the wires can't be placed back and it bothers you, try to cover the sharp area with wax. If this still doesn't work and you really can't stand it, call the office to come in and fix it.

Sometimes orthodontists will use metal ties, instead of color ties, to tie the wires to the brackets. The metal wires around the brackets may accidentally get loose, stick out, and cause irritation to your lips and cheeks. Try to tug the pokey wire back by using the end of a pencil eraser. If that is not possible, try to apply wax to it to relieve the irritation until your next appointment.

CHAPTER 9

AFTER ORTHODONTIC TREATMENT – ORTHODONTIC RETENTION

Now that you have a beautiful smile and all your teeth are straight and nice, you can't wait to ask your orthodontist to remove your braces. Your orthodontist then tells you that you need to wear retainers! What? Didn't you just work really hard for two years with braces and a bunch of "rubber bands?"

1. WHAT IS A RETAINER?

Retainers are the appliances that hold your teeth after braces treatment to ensure your teeth will maintain the straight position for a lifetime.

2. HOW MANY TYPES OF RETAINERS ARE THERE?

Some of my patients will ask me to give them "permanent "retainers. Most of the time they mean "fixed" retainers. There are two types of retainers: fixed and removable. Fixed retainers are glued in your mouth to hold your teeth. Removable retainers are removed and replaced into the mouth by patients. Which type of retainer is better? It depends on what kind of bite the patient's original bite was, and every patient is different. Your orthodontist should prescribe for you either a fixed or removable retainer, sometimes even both. There are also pros and cons for fixed vs removable retainers.

Fixed retainers:

Fixed retainers are usually a piece of metal bar glued behind your front teeth. Most of the fixed bar retainers are glued on the back of the lower anterior teeth for patients who had moderate to severe lower anterior crowding. You will also see lots of fixed retainer bars glued on the back of upper anterior teeth for patients with big gaps.

- Pros: Holds your teeth in place 24/7, so you do not have to wear removable retainers full time.

- Cons: Hard to floss in between teeth. Easily creates calculus build-up around the retainers and may cause long term periodontal problems. Only hold for the anterior teeth, and exclude the rest of other teeth. Hard to identify breakage until your teeth have shifted. They require repairs periodically and eventually need to be removed.

Removable retainers:

The most common removable retainers are clear, invisible plastic trays or acrylic Hawley retainers with a metal bar in the front. Patients are required to wear the removable retainers for a certain period of time in order to maintain the final result.

- Pros: They wrap around your teeth from front to the back so all your teeth will be held in place, not just the front teeth. Cleaning is easy so there are no periodontal concerns. Patients have full control to maintain the smile.

- Cons: Require patient's cooperation and dedication. The teeth will shift if patients are not wearing retainers as scheduled.

Your orthodontist will give you the recommendations in regards to which type of retainer will be the best for you.

3. HOW LONG DO I HAVE TO WEAR RETAINERS?

People ask me this question all the time. I typically ask my patients "how long do you want to have a perfect smile?" If your answer is "forever", then you should wear your retainers "forever." Our body does age and constantly changes every second. Therefore, you should commit to wearing retainers for a **LIFETIME** to ensure you have a beautiful smile for a lifetime. You will start by wearing retainers full time every night to every other night, and gradually go to one night a week for the rest of your life. Wearing retainers for your lifetime will be the best insurance and cheapest investment for you to ensure you keep your perfect, beautiful smile for a lifetime.

4. WHAT IF I LOSE OR BREAK MY RETAINERS?

Please call your orthodontic office to obtain new retainers. I consider it an **EMERGENCY!** It is cheaper to get a new set of retainers than to get braces again since your teeth will shift without retainers. Don't wait and see. Be proactive to protect your perfect smile.

5. HOW DO I CLEAN MY RETAINERS?

Rule #1: Always clean your retainers and your teeth prior to wearing your retainers. Never wear your retainers with dirty teeth: they will stain your retainers.

Rule #2: Use regular to cold temperature water to clean your retainers. Never clean your retainers with hot water. Hot water will distort your retainers.

Rule #3: Use liquid soap or mouth rinse to clean your retainers with a tooth brush. Avoid frequent use of toothpaste since it contains abrasive particles that will wear down your retainers.

CHAPTER 10

FINAL WORDS-MY SECRET RECIPES FOR SUCCESSFUL ORTHODONTIC TREATMENT

Orthodontic treatment has been commoditized. Orthodontic treatment should be perceived as a medical treatment, not a "product" to straighten your smile, since orthodontist's experience and level of skills do vary. A common misconception is that a beautiful smile can be achieved at any orthodontist's office as long as it is nearby and cheap. However, as parents, we should want the absolute best for our children and their oral health.

Orthodontic treatment is like cooking. It is an art and has to be customized to the individual palate! Each chef may have their favorite ingredients and secret sauces to create delicious dishes. Also, their most popular dish may taste like heaven to Mary, but may not be appreciated by John. Some chefs will only offer the freshest ingredients and add condiments to the dishes with artistic creativity, while others will make everything simple and use the most inexpensive ingredients. Which chef would you prefer to cook for you? Please allow me to share my secret recipes that contribute to our patients' successful orthodontic treatment:

PRIOR TO YOUR ORTHODONTIC TREATMENT: CHOOSING THE RIGHT ORTHODONTIST FOR YOU

Recipe #1: Do your research to find reputable orthodontists in your area.

There are several ways to find your future orthodontist. The most common and convenient way is to google orthodontists in your city. I must warn you to proceed with caution when using Internet search methods. The most popular orthodontists on Google do not always equal the best orthodontists. These orthodontists with high visibility may be the best Internet marketers at attracting new patients, while some of the best orthodontists in town may not have big budgets to spend on marketing.

Another good way to search for your orthodontist will be by word-of-mouth from your friends, family members, colleagues and your family dentists. You typically cannot go wrong with word- of-mouth referrals. My patients often find me through their dentists, since I treat a lot of dentists' children. If these dentists are willing to send their children to the orthodontist for treatment, you know the orthodontist should be trustworthy!

I would recommend you find a couple of orthodontists' names in your area, and make consultation appointments with the offices. Trust your gut feeling and see how the offices treat you while you visit them and make your best judgment.

Recipe #2: Do not choose your orthodontist because they are the cheapest!

I have emphasized this point a million times in my book. Money talks, I understand. Unless you cannot differentiate the value and care your orthodontist can offer, you can then definitely opt for the cheaper orthodontist. However, if you know that one of the orthodontists you like costs a little more due to the superior value and care they can offer, stay with them as it is worth paying them a little bit extra! Trust me, it is you and/or your children's face and smile for a lifetime, so do not let your checkbook dictate what should be your best decision.

Recipe #3: Our patients love us! We love our patients and their parents. We let our patients know how much we adore

and cherish our relationship with their family on a regular basis.

Do you love your orthodontist and the team? Every orthodontic treatment will take about eighteen to twenty-four months, and you will see your orthodontist and their team every six to ten weeks. Other than seeing orthodontists, I can only think of going to my OBGYN's office that often while I was pregnant. Therefore, you must enjoy every visit with your orthodontist and the team. *You should feel like your orthodontist's office is like your second home!* Everybody should know your name and greet you warmly. A successful orthodontic treatment starts with a great relationship between you and your orthodontist's office.

DURING ORTHODONTIC TREATMENT

Recipe #1: Our patients have regular visits and adjustments with our offices.

We always remind our patients of their appointments through automatic text, phone calls or emails. Again, your teeth won't be straightened by just having braces or Invisalign®. Your braces and Invisalign® need to be constantly adjusted by your orthodontist. Most failed treatment results are attributed to the infrequent visits to an orthodontist's office. Remember, you are only "decorating" your teeth with braces or Invisalign® if you don't see your orthodontist for routine adjustments.

Recipe #2: We are constantly connecting with our patients and parents to make orthodontic treatment a part of their priorities.

Our lives are busy with school, homework, after school sports practice, music lessons, work, and grocery shopping. How do we have time to remember wearing elastics and headgear like we are supposed to? In our office, we constantly connect with our patients through emails, newsletters and social media. We share valuable tips for successful orthodontic treatment, and constantly remind them to wear their appliances when they are not seeing us.

Recipe #3: We provide positive, ultimate patient experience.

Orthodontic treatment is boring? Not in our office! We offer video games for our patients and siblings while they are in the office. There are numerous fun contests to participate in and win prizes. We have theme weeks like 'Hawaii luau' or 'PJ week' with doctors, staff and patients dressing up with lots of compliments, laughter and fun pictures taken. Patients enjoy patient appreciation days with free movies at local theaters where all their friends and family are invited. Our patients are competing for "Patient of the Month" to be featured in our newsletter. Again, orthodontic treatment can be fun and rewarding, not just a process to straighten your crooked teeth.

Recipe #4: Understand the concept of teamwork for successful orthodontic treatment.

Who is the superstar in the team that gives you a fabulous superstar smile at the end? You or your orthodontist and team? The answer is all. Often, parents place the success or failure of orthodontic treatment solely on the orthodontist and the orthodontic team. For the whole two year process, the patient will only visit an orthodontic office every six to ten weeks. For the rest of the time, the patient is responsible for eating properly (so as to not damage orthodontic appliances), cleaning appliances and teeth spotlessly, wearing elastics, and changing Invisalign® trays and headgear by following the doctor's instruction. The patient and parents make frequent appointments advised by the orthodontist, and visit their family dentist for checkups and cleanings every four to six months during the treatment. The orthodontist, the team, the patient and parents, and the family dentist are all the superstars and make the dream teamwork come true.

Recipe #5: We are the orthodontists and cheerleaders for your fabulous smiles!

I really enjoy the concept of "positive reinforcement" for my patients. It really works better than the "negative reinforcement" method. I used to be the "police" orthodontist during my earlier career stage. I would nag on patients about loose appliances, missing appointments and failing to wear elastics. It created this tension between the young patient, the parent and myself, and destroyed the pleasant experience we aim for during the orthodontic treatment. I now consider myself a cheerleader orthodontist! I will make fun of myself to "beg" them not to have loose appliances or to wear more elastics. I will encourage and reward them with positive words and make them believe in themselves so that they can stop breaking the appliances and be in charge of their treatment. I and my team will sing and dance for them when they are doing so well during the treatment. We celebrate every single success for our patients' wonderful progress and achievement.

AFTER FINISHING ORTHODONTIC TREATMENT

Recipe #1: Let your orthodontist "beautify" your smile.

Prior to or after removing orthodontic appliances, I often ask permission to "beautify" my patients' upper and lower six front teeth. I will use a disk to polish and smooth out the irregular edges of patients' front teeth. I advise patients that they may feel " ticklish" and may be a little bit sensitive, especially for the lower teeth, while I am beautifying their teeth. The process typically takes me less than five minutes, but the patients always exclaim "wow" for what the "touch-up" could do for their smiles and teeth. We call this procedure "enamoplasty"! It is artistic work for me to enhance our patient's smiles with ultimate, superior esthetics! Our patients just love it, and some of them keep asking me to do it over and over again.

Recipe #2: Enhance your fabulous smiles with teeth whitening.

Now you have a straight and perfect smile after braces, Invisalign® and enamoplasty. What more can we do to enhance your smile? Having a perfect, pearly white Hollywood smile is not a far-reached dream anymore!

After two years of orthodontic treatment to meet the deadline for Jennifer's big wedding day in June, Jennifer was very pleased to see her fabulous straight smile for her upcoming wedding photos. She had a perfect wedding gown from Vivian Westwood and flawless makeup ready for the photo shoot. While smiling in front of the mirror, she noticed her teeth were yellowish, like mustard, and her perfectly white wedding gown magnified her yellowish smile. Jennifer postponed the wedding photo shoots and desperately called me to see if there were any solutions to get rid of her yellow smile. I advised her to have in-office Zoom whitening with the proposal of $500. She was hesitant about the whitening cost at the beginning, considering she just spent thousands of dollars for her orthodontic treatment.

After calculating her expenses on her wedding, she realized how much she had spent for her perfect once-in-a-lifetime wedding: the perfect flower arrangements, bridal gown, and three course dinner with Grand Cru Champagne. She realized everything was almost perfect except for her yellow smile. She made the appointment with us immediately, hopping into my dental chair for a one-and-a-half hour appointment for Zoom Whitening. By the time she was done, her teeth were as perfectly white as her wedding gown. She was now a happy and confident bride, and after orthodontic treatment, considers Zoom whitening the best investment she ever made.

For slightly discolored teeth, I would recommend patients try over-the-counter bleaching strips, such as Crest Whitestrips. These are easy-to-use whitening strips applied across your teeth during sleep with a monthly cost of $30. This inexpensive method can get you some visible whitening effects for about four-shade improvements, depending on individual variation.

Recipe #3: Enhance your fabulous smiles with bondings, veneers or crowns.

Even with a straight smile after braces or Invisalign®, some patients will still need additional prosthetic work to complete the process. It is not uncommon to see patients with disproportionally small upper lateral incisors or pointed canines brought forward to replace congenitally missing lateral incisors. The look of these teeth will easily be enhanced by adding composite bonding materials, fake nail-sized veneers, or crown preparation at the surfaces of these teeth.

Composite bonding materials are tooth-colored adhesives dentists use to restore cavities. There are varied shades of composite to match your tooth color. You do need an artistic dentist who can meticulously match your tooth color and modify the shape and size of your front teeth. The cost per tooth is about $200-$500 and should last for a decade.

I recommend composite bonding for patients who need slight to moderate improvements for their tooth appearance and have a limited budget to spend on the dental work. To achieve "extreme makeover" results, veneers and crowns will be the magic wand to make your dream come true. Veneers are paper-thin porcelain laminates, similar to wood floor laminates. The cost of veneer per tooth ranges from $1000-$2000, and you typically need at least four to six as a set for your upper front teeth, which can end up being very pricey. The dentist removes poker-card thinned enamel from your teeth, an impression is taken, and you will have a temporary bonding applied back to your teeth. The lab will fabricate your veneers according to the impression and prescription of your dentist. Several weeks later, you will receive the final veneers and the delivery procedure takes about two hours. A well-done veneer looks natural and admirable, and it can usually last for 15 years and more. You really need a highly-skilled dentist to deliver these pricey cosmetic results.

I personally am not a big fan of using crowns for cosmetic reasons, since they are expensive and require the removal of significant tooth structures. A crown ranges from $700-$2000, and it can last more than 15 years. The materials of crowns do not differ too much, so patients will pay more for higher skilled and artistic dentists and the quality of lab. However, I will only have crowns done if there is absolutely no other option.

Recipe #4: Replace your missing teeth as soon as possible.

Right after finishing orthodontic treatment, all missing teeth will need to be replaced immediately. If not, your straight teeth may shift and your bite will be off down the road, and you will need orthodontic treatment again. Secondly, the bone at the missing tooth area will continue to decline, and you will need an expensive and extensive bone graft surgical procedure in the future. Thirdly, the roots adjacent to the missing teeth have the tendency to move toward the empty tooth site. We see this so often, even when patients wear their retainer faithfully. The teeth will shift because the roots shift, and patients who need dental implants will need orthodontic treatment again to reposition the roots.

The options are dental implants, bridges and removable dentures. The ultimate option will absolutely be dental implants, which is the standard care in dentistry. If you ask one hundred dentists what to have when it comes to replacing their own missing teeth, all the dentists will choose dental implants. The cost per dental implant is about $1500-$3000, and should last almost for a lifetime if done correctly with the right surgeons. I do emphasize "surgeons," such as periodontists and oral surgeons. If you are offered an implant for $1000, or by a non-surgeon specialist, I recommend you RUN AWAY as fast as you can. After the placement of dental implants, crowns will be needed to complete the implant restoration, which will be performed by your family dentist or prosthodontist. Again, an implant crown ranges from $700-$2000. In general, a complete dental implant surgery and crown restoration ranges from $2200-$5000. I know the price tag is high and scary, but it will be the best investment in your life!

Recipe #5: Recontour your gum with esthetic crown lengthening.

Now Mary's teeth are perfectly straight after two years of orthodontic treatment. I have "beautified" her front teeth, and she has done in-office tooth whitening. The smile is "almost perfect" but it just doesn't look even to Mary. "Something is just not right?" Mary said. When closely analyzing Mary's smile, I identified she had uneven shape in her gum at her upper front teeth, and the unevenness was even more obvious when she smiled. Because of her uneven gum line, some teeth appeared longer than others. Mary was referred to the periodontist, Dr. H. Dr. H recommended a periodontal procedure called esthetic crown lengthening. After getting Mary comfortable with some local anesthetics, Dr. H trimmed some of Mary's extra bone and tissue to even out the bone levels of her six front teeth. The procedure took about one hour, and the cost was around $2000-$4000. (Don't you think braces are way cheaper for two years of hard work?) Mary was surprised that it only took less than one hour. She experienced a little giddiness and minimal discomfort overnight. After one week, Mary went back to Dr. H for a post-operative checkup and suture removal, and was able to see the beautiful, even look of her gum. "What a transformation!" Mary exclaimed, "Now I really like my smile and I feel fabulous."

Recipe #6: We asked all our patients to wear their retainers for a lifetime.

Shame on some of the orthodontists in our field. I often hear patients need orthodontic treatment again because their orthodontist never mentioned the necessity of lifetime retainer wearing. Please listen carefully: you need to wear retainers for your lifetime if you want to maintain your fabulous superstar smiles. Every cellular element of our body changes every single second, and our teeth do shift regardless of whether you having braces or not. Retainers, again, will be your best "life insurance" to ensure your investment in orthodontic treatment can last for ages. I don't recommend having fixed retainers in a patient's mouth for a lifetime, since they may create potential hygiene and gum disease problems. I advise my patients to use removable retainers, clear plastic or Hawley retainers, occasionally – such as once a week during night time wear. I guarantee you will keep your fabulous superstar smiles for a lifetime if you follow my regimen.

Make sure to call your orthodontist's office immediately to replace any missing or broken retainers as it is considered an "emergency"! Do not just ignore it and "pray" that your teeth will not shift. Trust me; your teeth will shift without wearing retainers routinely! Your wisest investment is to replace your retainers at a fraction of the cost it would take to undergo orthodontic treatment again.

Recipe #7: Make sure to visit your family dentist every six months.

Realistically, you should have less dental problems such as decay and gum disease after orthodontic treatment, since your teeth are straight and easy to clean. However, please still see your dentist twice a year for early detection of any potential dental disease, if there is any. Often patients develop gum disease in their later life and the disease compromises the foundation of the teeth. You will start seeing your teeth shift even with frequent retainer wearing. Retainers can hardly hold periodontally-compromised teeth successfully. Also, if you happen to having missing teeth due to decay, gum disease or fractures, and you postpone replacing the missing teeth, your teeth will also start to shift toward the missing tooth space and change your occlusion. Seeing your family dentist will be perfect to prevent the entire potential problem from happening.

I hope you have enjoyed my secret recipes for using braces and Invisalign® for orthodontic treatment. They are all my best! Enjoy your fabulous, superstar smile journey with your orthodontic chef. Bon Appetit!

CHAPTER 11
(BONUS CHAPTER #1)

CELEBRITIES WEARING BRACES AND INVISALIGN®

BY KATIE FORTUNA

Not everybody is born with a Fabulous Superstar Smile! Many people will require braces at some point in their life. The following famous superstars chose to sport some hardware after they were all stars! This just goes to show that even the most seemingly perfect people need their smile perfected! From actors and musicians to athletes and even royals, fabulous superstar smiles are a trend that is sweeping the nation!

Here are some famous faces in braces!

Faith Hill – *Clear Braces* - Grammy Award-Winning Country Singer, known for her chart topping songs "This Kiss" and "Breathe." Faith wore braces as a teenager, but admittedly neglected to wear her retainer, so she needed them again as an adult!

Faye Dunaway – *Traditional Metal* - Academy Award-Winning Actress. Best known for "Bonnie and Clyde" and "Network." Faye had her braces put on when she was 61 years old! She admitted that sometimes your teeth just get away from you and she wanted to polish up her smile. When Faye had her braces removed, she also had veneers placed!

Miley Cyrus – *Traditional Metal* - American Singer and Actress. Known for "Hannah Montana" and "Wrecking Ball." Miley Cyrus had to have her braces removed before filming a season of "Hannah Montana" because the producers didn't believe that braces fit the character.

Tom Cruise – *Clear Braces* - American Actor. Known for "Top Gun," "Jerry Maguire," and the "Mission Impossible" franchise. Tom Cruise wore braces for a few months in 2002, just to fix the small imperfections in his teeth. Tom having braces on seemed to make braces "cool" again!

Kate Middleton – *Lingual Braces* – Duchess of Cambridge Princess Kate had lingual braces in order to fix the imperfections in her teeth. Reports claim that the princess did not want an "artificial" smile, but instead wanted her teeth to look "natural" so her treatment purposefully left some small imperfections.

Justin Bieber – *Invisalign®* – Canadian Singer/Songwriter, known for songs such as "Baby" and "What Do You Mean?" Justin was spotted wearing his invisible aligners to straighten his smile in 2010.

Beyoncé – *Traditional Braces* – Grammy Award-Winning Singer/Songwriter and Actress, known for "Crazy in Love" and "Single Ladies (Put a Ring on it)." Beyonce didn't actually require braces, but she wore them for one day in 2011 to show support for all of her young fans that wore braces, stating that even those with braces can have a beautiful smile!

Gwen Stefani – *Traditional Braces* – Grammy Award-Winning Singer Songwriter, Fashion Designer, and Actress, known for being a member of the rock band, No Doubt, a solo musical career, and being a judge on the hit television program "the Voice." Gwen started sporting braces in 1999 as a fashion decision! She claims she always wanted them as a child, but couldn't afford them, so she decided to put braces on as an adult!

Alyssa Milano – *Clear Braces* - American Actress known for "Melrose Place," and "Charmed." Alyssa stunned her fans in 2005 by sporting some hardware in her mouth! The actress has also been spotted in public wearing her retainer!

Nicholas Cage – *Traditional Braces* – Academy Award-Winning Actor known for "Leaving Las Vegas" and "National Treasure." Nick had braces on his lower teeth as an adult. He got his braces in between movies so that he could perfect his movie star smile.

Cristiano Ronaldo – *Clear Braces* – Professional Soccer Player, known for playing with the Portuguese National Team and Spanish Soccer Team Real Madrid. While playing in England for Manchester United, Cristiano wore braces to fix his crooked smile. Orthodontia also opened up a spot in Ronaldo's mouth for a dental implant to be placed where his upper right lateral incisor should have been.

Dwight Howard – *Traditional Braces* – Professional Basketball Player, known for playing with the Orlando Magic, the Los Angeles Lakers, and the Houston Rockets. Dwight had braces from age 14 to age 19, when he was signed in the NBA Draft by the Orlando Magic. He admits that he hated them at first, but came to love having braces after he was used to them.

Niall Horan – *Clear Braces* – Member of the British Pop Group, *One Direction*, known for "What Makes you Beautiful" and "Story of My Life." Niall had braces put on his teeth in 2011 when his band, One Direction, was skyrocketing to superstardom.

Emma Watson – *Traditional Braces* – British Actress known for the "Harry Potter" franchise and "the Perks of Being a Wallflower." Emma wore braces for only 4 months! Because she had braces on for such a short time, she was able to have all of her orthodontic work done between the 2nd and 3rd Harry Potter Movies!

Nelson Cruz – *Clear Braces* – Professional Baseball Player, known for playing for the Texas Rangers and the Seattle Mariners. Nelson was spotted in 2012 wearing braces while on the field playing with the Texas Rangers.

Fantasia Barrino – *Clear Braces* – American R&B Singer, known for winning season 3 of American Idol. The American Idol winner wore braces for about one year in 2008 after winning the hit TV show in 2004. Having a straight smile seems to have been of the utmost importance for the singer, because she was spotted in 2012 wearing her retainers!

Dakota Fanning – *Clear Braces* – American Actress known for "I Am Sam" and the "Twilight" franchise. Dakota Fanning has a long history of dental work! Starting at age 10 she got her first set of braces, and even had to have teeth pulled, wear a headgear, and even have dental surgery! By her 14th birthday, Dakota had movie star caliber teeth! The amazing part is that Dakota never had braces on in any of her movie roles as a child!

Princess Eugenie of York – *Traditional Braces* – Daughter of Prince Andrew of York, Grandchild of Queen Elizabeth II. Princess Eugenie wore braces for 2 years from 2007 to 2009 to ensure that her smile was of Royal Caliber!

Katherine Heigl – *Invisalign®* – Emmy Award-Winning Actress known for "Grey's Anatomy" and "27 Dresses." Katherine never really had interest in braces until she became engaged. The actress said she wanted to fix her smile for her engagement photos!

Danny Glover – *Clear Braces* – American Actor known for "Lethal Weapon" and "Angels in the Outfield." Danny was wearing braces while filming the movie "Shooter" and many people claim that his voice was altered with a lisp because of his orthodontia!

Tyra Banks – *Invisalign®* – American Supermodel and TV Personality, known for being a Victoria's Secret "Angel," as well as on the TV Shows "America's Next Top Model" and "the Tyra Banks Show." Tyra wore braces for two-and-a-half years to obtain her supermodel smile

Brett Favre – *Clear Braces* – American Football Quarterback, known for winning the Super Bowl XXXI with the Green Bay Packers. Brett braved orthodontia while throwing touchdowns for the Green Bay Packers!

Estelle – *Clear Braces* – Grammy Award-Winning British Singer/Songwriter known for "American Boy" and "Thank You." Estelle had braces placed in 2008. She claims she had them because she wanted to win a Grammy and didn't want people to comment on her teeth if she got to accept the award.

About Katie Fortuna

Professional Relations Coordinator – Significance Dental Specialists

Katie was born in Providence, Rhode Island. At the age of 12, her family moved to Reno, NV which is where she completed her K-12 education. She graduated from the University of Nevada, Las Vegas with a Bachelor's degree in Psychology. After graduation,she began working for Significance Dental Specialists' orthodontic team as a scheduling coordinator. Within a year, her job title shifted and she now work as a Professional Relations Coordinator. She absolutely loves that her job allows her to be creative and forge meaningful personal and professional relationships with co-workers as well as employees and doctors from dental offices throughout the Las Vegas Valley.

Katie's hobbies include playing music, teaching music and choreography to local band programs, going to various Broadway and philharmonic performances, and proudly supporting the U.S. Men's and Women's National Soccer Teams, as well as Arsenal FC in the English Premier League.

You can connect with Katie at significancekatie@hotmail.com

CHAPTER 12
(BONUS CHAPTER #2)

BRACES FRIENDLY RECIPES

Patients and their parents often ask me what to eat during orthodontic treatment. Other than Invisalign® patients, who literally have no restriction in food selection, it can be a challenging and frustrating thing for our braces patients or the parents when it comes to lunch and dinner time.

I am a good orthodontist, but I am horrible when it comes to the real "women's world" - the kitchen! I have no creativity at all for cooking! Fortunately, I have a multi-talented team who not only excel in their profession at dentistry, but also are excellent home chefs.

Andi Irons has been our hygienist for almost ten years. Andi's husband, Larry, is a trained Chef from a well known Las Vegas culinary school, Le Cordon Bleu. Larry had his own catering company for years and published an interactive video cook book, *The Home Chef*. When I asked for braces-friendly recipes, Andi and Larry were very generous and willing to contribute some of their best recipes for our orthodontic patients.

Sarah Reyes is our Patient Care Coordinator, and absolutely adored by our patients. While I was desperately asking for braces-friendly recipes, I realized Sarah had a passion for cooking, and "fed" three of her boys successfully when they had braces.

In this bonus chapter, you will find a variety of creative ideas for daily cooking and even desserts. They are not only braces-friendly, but also super delicious! These recipes are great for both adults and children. While looking for fabulous superstar smiles, you can absolutely enjoy delicious meals and live a fabulous lifestyle.

Who says having braces is boring and miserable? They are so WRONG!

Quinoa (pronounced **KEEN-wah**) is a South American grain which was a staple of the ancient Incas. It contains more protein than any other grain, and is used extensively in salads, soups, or like rice, as a side dish.

QUINOA & VEGETABLE SALAD

By Our Hygienist and her Home Chef hubby:
Andi and Larry Irons

1 Cup Quinoa, rinsed well

2 Cups Water

½ tsp Turmeric

1 Cup Carrot, shredded

½ Cup Celery, small dice

1 Small Red Bell Pepper, small dice

2 Fresh Roma Tomatoes, chopped

1 – 14oz Can "No Salt Added" Corn

1 Jalapeno, ribs & seeds removed & minced

2 Green Onions, sliced thin, both green & white parts

½ Cup Pumpkin Seeds, toasted

2 TBS Sunflower Seeds, toasted

3 oz Fresh Lemon Juice

3 TBS Low-Sodium Tamari Soy Sauce

Sea Salt & Fresh Ground Black Pepper, to taste

1. Place the rinsed quinoa in a soup pot (with no liquid) and cook over medium heat, stirring frequently until it turns golden brown.

2. Turn the heat to high, add 2 cups water and the turmeric to quinoa and bring to a boil. Stir, cover, turn heat to low and simmer 12 – 15 minutes until all water is absorbed. Remove pot from heat and let stand uncovered.

3. Mix together carrots, celery, red bell pepper, tomato, corn, jalapeno, green onions, pumpkin seeds and sunflower seeds. Add this mixture to the quinoa and mix gently.

4. In a small bowl, whisk together the lemon juice and tamari. Add this to the quinoa mixture and toss. Chill in refrigerator for 30 minutes or up to 3 hours. Chill salad plates in refrigerator at the same time.

5. Season to taste with sea salt and fresh ground black pepper. Put a whole butter lettuce leaf on a chilled salad plate or bowl and put 2 or 3 serving-spoon spoonfuls on lettuce. Garnish with a sprig or two of cilantro and serve.

Yield: 6 servings

The term cuisson (KWEE-sohn) means a sauce made from a poaching liquid.

POACHED HALIBUT WITH MUSTARD-CREAM CUISSON

By Our Hygienist and her Home Chef hubby:
Andi and Larry Irons

2 Quarts Water

1 Bay Leaf

12 Black Peppercorns

3 Sprigs Fresh Dill

2 TBS Lemon Juice

6 – 6 oz Halibut Steaks

2 TBS Dijon Style Mustard

1 Pint Heavy Cream

1 TBS Unsalted Butter

Salt, to taste

White Pepper, to taste

1 TBS Fresh Dill, minced

1. Put the water in a large Dutch oven. Add the bay leaf, peppercorns, fresh dill and lemon juice and bring to a gentle simmer. Simmer 10 minutes.

2. Add the halibut steaks and cook 10 minutes. Remove from poaching liquid and keep warm.

3. Pour the poaching liquid through a fine strainer and keep 2 cups. Add the 2 cups to a small saucepan over medium heat and stir in the mustard, stirring constantly until it is completely incorporated. Whisk in the heavy cream and bring to a gentle simmer. Let this cook, stirring occasionally, until reduced by half.

4. Whisk in the butter and season to taste with salt and white pepper.

5. Place halibut steaks on plates and top with a little mustard-cream sauce. Sprinkle on a little minced dill and serve.

Yield: 6 servings

Some think cheddar cheese was invented in Wisconsin, but the truth is it was invented in the English village of Cheddar sometime around 1170. There is no protected designation of origin for cheddar, so even though it is made much differently today and tastes much different today, no matter where it is made and by what process, it can be called cheddar. In the U.S., Wisconsin produces the most cheddar.

WISCONSIN MEAT LOAF

By Our Hygienist and her Home Chef hubby:
Andi and Larry Irons

2 lbs Ground Chuck

½ Red Onion, cut small dice

2 Cloves Garlic, minced

2 Eggs, beaten

½ Cup Fine Bread Crumbs

2 TBS Tomato Paste

2 Cups Tomato Sauce

1½ tsp Salt

¼ tsp Black Pepper

1 tsp Oregano

3 Cups Wisconsin Cheddar Cheese, shredded

3 oz Cheddar Cheese, cut in 2-inch long by ½ -inch wide strips

½ Cup Tomato Sauce

½ Cup Parsley, chopped

1. In a large bowl, combine all ingredients, except cheddar. Mix well. Lay on parchment paper and shape into a square, 12"x12".

2. Cover with cheddar leaving a 1-inch border around the entire square. Roll like a jellyroll and press down on ends pinching to seal tightly. Place on a baking sheet or shallow pan and bake for 1¼ hours.

3. Remove from oven and shut door to keep in heat. Add the strips of cheese across entire loaf, top with ½ cup tomato sauce and put back in the oven and bake another 5 minutes

4. To serve, slice into 1-inch thick slices and sprinkle on chopped parsley. Serve with mashed potatoes and green beans, if desired.

Yield: 8 servings

Pad Thai is made with tamarind, which is a paste that smells and tastes a bit like molasses. Tamarind means "date of India", and is used in many Asian dishes. It is used to make Worcestershire sauce, which was invented by two Britons named Lea & Perrins.

PAD THAI

By Our Hygienist and her Home Chef hubby:
Andi and Larry Irons

1 Package Rice Noodles (also known as rice sticks)

1 Cup Tamarind, soaked in ¾ cup boiling water and strained

2 TBS Peanut Oil, divided

24 Small Shrimp, deveined

1 Shallot, minced

2 Cloves Garlic, smashed and minced

3 Egg Yolks, beaten

7 - 8 Dried Shrimp, chopped very fine

2 TBS Daikon Radish, minced

3 TBS Fish Sauce

3 TBS Sugar

1 tsp Rice Wine Vinegar

1 tsp Cayenne

¼ Cup Bean Sprouts

2 Green Onions, green part only, cut small on bias

4 TBS Peanuts, chopped rough

2 TBS Cilantro, chopped

Lime Juice, as needed

1. Heat 2 quarts water to 150°F. Place rice noodles in bowl large enough to accommodate them all and pour hot water over. Let sit 20 minutes.

2. Soak tamarind in ¾ cup boiling water until it becomes soft. Strain as much pulp as possible through a fine sieve and set aside. Heat 1 TBS peanut oil in a non-stick skillet to very hot and cook shrimp, turning constantly until they begin to caramelize slightly on the outside and turn pink elsewhere. Set aside

3. Remove pan from heat and add 1 TBS peanut oil. Add shallots and garlic, turn heat back to medium and cook, stirring constantly.

4. Add eggs yolks and mix well with shallots and garlic, cooking about 3 minutes. Add dried shrimp, daikon, noodles, fish sauce, sugar, rice vinegar and cayenne. Turn heat to high and cook, stirring constantly for 2 - 3 minutes.

5. Add tamarind, cooked shrimp, bean sprouts and green onions. Cook 2 minutes tossing constantly. Garnish with chopped peanuts, cilantro and lime juice.

Yield: 6 servings

There are literally hundreds of species of scallops around the world, but the top three in the U.S. are bay scallops; Japanese sea scallops; and North Atlantic sea scallops.

North Atlantic sea scallops are the largest of the three, and are sold 10/40 count per pound. (The bigger the number, the fewer there are to a pound.)

BACON WRAPPED SEA SCALLOPS

By Our Hygienist and her Home Chef hubby:
Andi and Larry Irons

18 North Atlantic Sea Scallops

18 Slices Apple-Wood Smoked Bacon

Toothpicks

1. Preheat Broiler. Rinse scallops and pat dry with paper towels.

2. Wrap each scallop with 1 slice of bacon. Secure with toothpicks.

3. Place on baking pan and place baking pan about 6-inches below broiler flame. Broil 6 - 10 minutes per side, or until bacon is cooked and starting to get crisp.

4. Remove from oven and serve with tartar sauce or horseradish sauce if desired.

Yield: 6 servings, 3 to a serving

Even those who don't like vegetables will like this and most will not believe it is made with vegetables. Of course the cream cheese has something to do with it. This dip is especially good on wheat thins, celery sticks and toasted pita bread. It also makes a good sandwich spread when topped with onions, sliced tomatoes, sliced olives and lettuce.

ROASTED VEGETABLE SPREAD

By Our Hygienist and her Home Chef hubby:
Andi and Larry Irons

1 Red Bell Pepper, seeded and cut in chunks

1 Sweet Yellow Onion, sliced into rings

4 Cloves Garlic, crushed

1 Zucchini, sliced

1 TBS Olive Oil

8 oz Cream Cheese

Kosher Salt, to taste

Freshly Ground Black Pepper, to taste

Crackers or Crudités

1. Preheat oven to 400°F. Place the bell pepper, onion, garlic, zucchini, and olive oil in a medium mixing bowl and toss until the vegetables are coated. Spread the vegetables evenly on sheet pan lined with foil and place to the oven. Roast, tossing occasionally, until they are soft, about 45 minutes.

2. Remove from the oven and place the red bell peppers in a baggie and seal tightly. Let sit 20 minutes, then remove skin. Let peppers and other vegetables cool completely.

3. Place the vegetables in the bowl of a food processor along with the cream cheese and process until well combined, but not completely smooth.

4. Taste and season with salt and pepper. Serve with crackers or even crudités. Store in the refrigerator in an airtight container for up to 1 week.

<u>Yield</u>: about 1½ cups

CHICKEN AND SUN DRIED TOMATO PASTA

By Our Patient Care Coordinator, Sarah Reyes

2 TBS. minced garlic

1 jar of sun dried tomatoes in oil

3 large boneless, skinless chicken breasts cut into small pieces

Pinch of salt

Dash of paprika to taste

1 cup of Half and Half or heavy cream

Shredded mozzarella cheese (about a cup or so)

½ cup of parmesan cheese

Penne pasta or any pasta of your choice

Dried basil, Italian seasoning, crushed red pepper flakes, salt

Reserve a little bit of your pasta water to add to the sauce

While the pasta is cooking, drain the tomatoes from the oil and chop small. Save a little oil to sautee the garlic and red pepper flakes. Add the chicken and sautee till no longer pink. Sprinkle with all the seasonings. Set chicken aside. Add the Half and Half and cheese and bring to a boil, add reserved water if cheese mix is too thick. Bring to a boil then add in the cooked pasta and serve.

Yield: 4 servings

EASY BREADSTICKS

By Our Patient Care Coordinator, Sarah Reyes

1 can of pizza crust (I use Pillsbury)

Melted butter

Mozzarella cheese

Parmesan cheese

Dried basil and garlic salt

1. Preheat oven to 425°F.

2. Unroll pizza crust and brush with butter

3. Sprinkle cheese and spices on top

4. Cut dough lengthwise into strips, then cut those strips in half

5. Don't separate the strips

6. Bake for 10 minutes or until golden brown

7. Serve warm

Yield: 12 servings

SESAME PINEAPPLE CHICKEN

By Our Patient Care Coordinator, Sarah Reyes

1 TBS. oil (I use sesame oil)

1 lb. boneless, skinless chicken breast or thigh

2 cups sugar snap peas

1 large red bell pepper

3 cloves of minced garlic

2 cups of fresh or canned pineapple chunks

¼ cup Asian sesame dressing of your choice

1 TBS. lite soy sauce

2 green onions chopped

Heat oil in a large skillet. Add chicken, peas, peppers, and garlic. Cook until chicken is done.

Add pineapple and cook for 2 minutes or so. Stir in combined dressing and soy sauce. Remove from heat, stir in onions and serve.

My suggestion is to serve with white rice or fried rice.

Yield: 4 servings

PUMPKIN CAKE

By Our Patient Care Coordinator, Sarah Reyes

Ingredients for the cake:

4 eggs

1 cup oil

1 16 oz can of Pumpkin (like Libby's)

1 2/3 cups of sugar

2 cups of flour

2 tsp. baking powder

1 tsp. baking soda

3 tsp. Cinnamon

1 tsp. salt

½ tsp. nutmeg

¼ tsp. ground cloves

Ingredients for the frosting:

8 oz of softened cream cheese

½ cup of softened butter

2 tsp. vanilla extract

2 cups of powdered sugar

Add milk to desired thickness and taste

Mix all of the cake ingredients together and pour into a greased glass baking dish (9 x 13) bake at 350°F for about 25 min. Cool before frosting.

Yield: 15 servings

Shortcake was a term used in the 15th Century to describe a bread or biscuit made crisp from the use of fat. When strawberries are in season, April – June, there is nothing better than strawberry shortcake, especially when you make the shortcakes.

STRAWBERRY SHORTCAKE

By Our Hygienist and her Home Chef hubby:
Andi and Larry Irons

2 Cups All Purpose Flour

¼ Cup Sugar

1 TBS Baking Powder

Zest of ½ Lemon, finely minced

¼ tsp Nutmeg

2 oz Butter, cold and cut into small pieces

1 Cup Buttermilk

Sugar, as needed

1½ pints Strawberries, hulls removed and sliced

¼ Cup Sugar (or more)

1 pint Sweetened Whipped Cream

1. Prepare the strawberries by removing the hulls and slicing into ¼ inch thick slices. Cover with the ¼ cup (or more) of sugar and let sit. Stir occasionally.

2. In a food processor combine the flour, ¼-cup sugar, baking powder, nutmeg and lemon zest and just pulse to combine. DON'T OVER PROCESS! Add the cold butter pieces steadily until the mixture looks like corn meal.

3. Remove to a large bowl and add the buttermilk, saving 2 TBS. Mix with your hands until a firm dough forms. It will be sticky. Line a sheet pan or cookie sheet with parchment paper and spray with vegetable cooking spray.

4. Make like snowballs, but don't compress tight. Each dough ball should be about 4 inches in diameter. Brush with a little buttermilk and sprinkle with sugar. Bake about 20 minutes at 350°F, or until very lightly browned.

5. To serve, split biscuits in half and top with strawberries. Be sure to include some of the juice. Add a big dollop of sweetened whipped cream and top with the other biscuit half.

Yield: 8 servings

LEMON-BLUEBERRY BUNDT CAKE

By Our Hygienist and her Home Chef hubby:
Andi and Larry Irons

Cooking Spray

2 TBS Granulated Sugar

3 Cups Flour (about 13 1/2 ounces)

1½ tsp Baking Powder

½ tsp Baking Soda

¼ tsp Salt

1 3/4 Cups Granulated Sugar

¼ Cup Butter, softened

1 TBS Lemon Zest, grated

4 Eggs

½ tsp Vanilla

16 oz Sour Cream

2 Cups Fresh Blueberries

To Make the Glaze:

1 Cup Powdered Sugar

3 TBS Fresh Lemon Juice

1. Preheat oven to 350°F.

2. Coat a 12-cup Bundt pan with cooking spray; dust with 2 tablespoons granulated sugar. Set aside.

3. Lightly spoon flour into dry measuring cups; level with a knife. Combine flour, baking powder, baking soda, and salt, stirring with a whisk.

4. Place 1¾ cups granulated sugar, butter, and rind in a large bowl; beat with a mixer at medium speed until well blended (about 2 minutes). Add eggs, 1 at a time, beating well after each addition (about 4 minutes total). Beat in vanilla and sour cream. Add flour mixture; beat at medium speed just until combined. Gently fold in blueberries. Spoon batter into prepared pan.

5. Bake 1 hour or until a wooden pick inserted in the center comes out clean. Cool in pan 15 minutes on a wire rack; remove from pan. Cool completely on wire rack.

6. To prepare glaze, combine powdered sugar and lemon juice, stirring well with a whisk. Drizzle over cooled cake.

Yield: 10 – 12 slices

About Andi Irons

Dental Hygienist at Significance Dental Specialists

A LOT OF IRONS IN THE FIRE!

I'll start in 1996 when I met my husband Larry Irons in Sparks, Nevada. Life circumstances had brought us to live next door to each other – we were both single at the time. We would joke with friends saying we had a 5,000 sq ft home on 2 acres. Or we would say we have one northern winter house, and a southern summer house. In actuality one house was 3000 sq ft which was located north of the other house which was 2000 sq ft. Eventually Larry could say he "married the girl next door". We sold both homes and moved to Las Vegas in July 1998.

We kept busy with a myriad of small entrepreneurial adventures, but the one thing I've always wanted to do was to be a dental hygienist. I already had a BA in biology, however, my science courses were beyond the seven-year limitation to enroll in the dental hygiene program at the College of Southern Nevada. So I took the time to refresh these courses – which was not difficult to me. I enrolled in the dental hygiene program and was accepted. I can honestly say this was the most demanding schooling I had ever endured! I graduated first in my class in 2006.

On another note, Larry had always been interested in cooking. He says his cooking was inspired by his grandma, who held him on her hip when he was four years old and let him cook his own eggs. Grandma owned the "Dew Drop Inn" in Reno, Nevada. After having a radio career over 30 years, which spanned nationwide, he saw an ad for Le Cordon Bleu College of Culinary Arts in Las Vegas. He checked out the school and really wanted to attend. He also graduated first in his class in 2005.

I have been working with Dr. Allen Huang since graduating dental hygiene school in 2006. I became so involved in the dental hygiene profession on the local and state level, the state organization – Nevada Dental Hygienists' Association – asked me to be the executive director. I've been in the administrative end of organizations since graduating high school working for the California Society of Anesthesiologists for 17 years, and am currently the executive director of the California Society of Physical Medicine and Rehabilitation since the year 2000.

So I was a good fit to oversee the statewide dental hygiene organization. Having experience with websites, I also fit the bill as the webmaster for the Nevada Dental Hygienists' Association, the Southern Nevada Dental Hygienists' Association, and the Northern Nevada Dental Hygienists' Association. Some of my duties are to design seminar brochures, eblast, batch fax, upload to the website, maintain registrations, continuing education certificates, etc. The list is too lengthy to include here. Then there are the board meetings for these organizations.

And did I mention I do all of this too for the Sigma Phi Alpha Beta Beta Beta chapter – which is the national dental hygiene honor society? And duplicate these efforts with the California Society of Physical Medicine and Rehabilitation organization too!

Many people have asked when I get any sleep. Sometimes it's difficult when there are multiple events taking place at nearly the same time. Larry is very supportive of all my activities and involvement. Who can say that their husband fixes meals and packs their lunch everyday when going to work. I smile at some of my classmates, who are a lot younger than I, when they say they are exhausted after working a three-day week! Hah! I am probably fifteen years older and work five days a week.

In my "spare" time I LOVE to pamper my children. My two children actually have four legs each. I've had Italian Greyhounds since 1993. At one time I had three dogs, three cats, and two macaws. Yes, it was a zoo. I've now settled in to only having two very spoiled dogs.

My newest venture which I am on the brink of starting is to educate staff/offices in infection control and OSHA standards. Being my name is Andi Irons, I guess you can say I have a "lot of irons in the fire!"

You can connect with Andi at andiironsrdh@cox.net

About Sarah Reyes
Patient Care Coordinator at Significance Orthodontics

I was born and raised in La Crescenta, California. I am the oldest daughter of three and I have two younger sisters who are more like best friends to me. I am a proud mother of three great boys. My oldest son, Anthony, is in college and has obtained three associate degrees in English, Humanities, and communication arts and is now going for his Bachelor's in English. This has been his passion to be an educator as far back as elementary school and I am so very proud. Alexander, my middle son, who is also in college is working on a degree in Business and will also study Graphic design. My youngest son, Christian, is in his first year of high school.

As my kids started getting older, I wanted to do something better with my life and start a career rather than different odd jobs here and there, mostly in retail and elderly care, so I decided to go into the dental field. I graduated from Concorde Career College in 2007 as a Dental Assistant and I have been working in the Orthodontic field since 2006. I enjoy what I do and working in Ortho is my passion. I enjoy it because of the genuine relationships I have built with my patients and families over the years.

I have many hobbies, all of them include spending time with my friends and family such as camping, outdoor activities, shopping, music, art, and my most favorite hobby of all is cooking. I search recipes for ideas and then take it and create something all my own, all together different. I get excited for my family to try new things that I have created in the kitchen.

You can connect with Sarah at: Sarahreyes76@yahoo.com.

www.ingramcontent.com/pod-product-compliance
Lightning Source LLC
Chambersburg PA
CBHW050236270326
41914CB00034BA/1945/J